Bar code: 383

## DATE DUE    #383

| | | | |
|---|---|---|---|
| | | | |
| | | | |
| | | | |
| | | | |
| | | | |
| | | | |
| | | | |
| | | | |
| | | | |
| | | | |

# strongerthancancer

Treasured Insights from the Hearts and
Homes of Families Fighting Cancer

BY CONNIE PAYTON

Edited by Dan Zadra with Debbie Cottrell
Designed by Kobi Yamada and Steve Potter

Published by Compendium, Inc.

## ACKNOWLEDGEMENTS

My heartfelt thanks to everyone who helped with this book, with special thanks to my parents, Issac and Rebia Norwood; to Walter's mom, Alyne Payton; to my late grandmother, Rosalie Barnes; to my tireless business manager, Kelly Woods; to Miss Luna; to Linda Conley; to all my friends and family (too many to name you all, but thank you for always being there); and to Jarrett and Brittney, you are the best thing that ever happened to Dad and my reason for being, please know that you are deeply loved and appreciated.

For aiding in the collection of these submissions, sincere thanks to: Cancer Treatment Centers of America (Jack Moore, Sheri Ziemann, Emily Breuker); Cancer Treatment Research Foundation (Fern Ingber, Alicia Stephenson); Cherie Chamness Foundation; Education Center for Prostate Cancer Patients; Facing Our Risk of Cancer Empowered; Healing Journeys; Jo's Trust; Johns Hopkins Breast Center; Kaiser Hospital-Santa Clara; Link To Life Newsletter (Cheryl Caleca); Magnet Communications (Jennifer Pfahler, Samantha Schnurr and Katie Goss); Mothers Supporting Daughters with Breast Cancer; National Alliance of Breast Cancer; National Brain Tumor Foundation; Betty Osborn; Run For Life; Taking The Fear Out Of Cancer; Young Survival; WA Practice Kindness, Seniors (Betty Kieler and friends)

Printed in Hong Kong

Love cures people, both the ones who give it, and the ones who receive it.

—DR. KARL MENNINGER

# foreword

In 1999, cancer took Walter Payton in the prime of his life. Shock and sadness enveloped the city of Chicago, and millions throughout the country stopped to mourn number 34—the legendary running back of the Chicago Bears. Walter was nicknamed "Sweetness," not for his athletic prowess or talent, but for his extraordinary kindness and character. Losing one so strong, so brave, so admired was a stark reminder that cancer plays no favorites.

But through it all, Walter and his family were never defeated. We recall how his courageous wife, Connie, and her children, Jarrett and Brittney, fought, laughed, loved, cried and dreamed right alongside with him. It's with that same passion that Connie Payton now leads the Walter Payton Cancer Fund (WPCF). Under the auspices of the Cancer Treatment Research Foundation (CTRF), the Walter Payton Cancer Fund supports cancer research for the innovative use of conventional treatments like chemotherapy and radiation, as well as for the best science-based complementary medicine. The goal is to provide cancer patients with the opportunity to live longer, more fruitful lives.

In writing this book, Connie brings cancer patients and their loved ones some of the much-needed advice she searched for during her own husband's illness. After reading countless books, Connie realized that some of the wisest advice for fighting cancer came, not just from medical experts, but straight from the hearts and homes of everyday friends and family. Combined with Connie's open-hearted, all-embracing style, this book is a true work of heart—a unique voice for the role of friends and family in the fight against cancer.

We are grateful to Cancer Treatment Centers of America (CTCA) for supporting this important book and generously underwriting daily operations for the Walter Payton Cancer Fund. CTCA helped provide the Payton family with hope, comfort and dignity, integrating medical expertise with innovative treatment options that were not easy to find. With CTCA's support, we can ensure that all proceeds from this book, as well as every dollar donated to the WPCF, go directly to breakthrough cancer research.

Enjoy this book and, as you do, I hope you will join me in thanking the Payton family—Connie, Jarrett and Brittney—for opening their hearts and sharing their intimate thoughts about their ongoing battle against this disease. The Paytons are living proof that together, we really *are* stronger than cancer.

*Fern K Ingber*

— Fern Ingber, President
Cancer Treatment Research Foundation

# introduction

We are winning the war on cancer, that's for sure. Times, treatments, and diagnoses are all improving as we speak. Almost every week brings news of a promising insight or advancement.

One of the biggest reasons we are winning is that we are no longer fighting fair. We have learned from long experience that ganging up on cancer is the surest way to beat it. Cancer is a bully and we are treating it as such.

Thanks to advancements in information technology, thousands of cancer researchers, doctors, and caregivers are swiftly combining the best of what we've learned. At Cancer Treatment Centers of America, one of the most important things we've learned is that we can't just fight cancer on a single front, we must attack and win on all three: Mind, Body and Spirit.

One of the most important fronts, of course, is the home front. This book shows the astonishing power of everyday friends and family in the war against cancer.

If you, or a friend, or loved one has recently been diagnosed, be assured that you are never helpless, and you are never fighting alone. As the people featured in this book attest, cancer is strong—but when all of us combine our love, faith, hope, energy and expertise—we are stronger.

*Connie Payton*

Connie Payton,
Chairman
Walter Payton Cancer Fund

Surround yourself
with people who
believe you can!

—JARRETT PAYTON

I am here.  Let's heal together.
**—A Friend**

These words helped see me through seven months of chemo: "When it hurts to look back, and you're scared to look ahead, look beside you—your best friend will be there."
**—VICKY GUNDLACH**

The day I went in for breast cancer surgery, my husband did the most wonderful thing.  Knowing it would be a long day, he purchased a big basket of get-well cards and colored pens and got together with our family and friends.  Everyone colored, or altered the words on the cards, and then decided which card I should open each day of my recovery.  For weeks after my surgery, I had something new to open every day and it reminded me how lucky I was to have such a great support group.
**—DIANE OBERQUELL**

When you think you can't take any more, hold out your hand—an angel will always come through to support you.  Believe!  Believe!  Believe!  You don't have to go through this alone.
**—STEPHANIE STULL**

"I couldn't have cancer! Everyone in my family lives to 95 to 100 years of age!" Just like many people, I was shocked with the diagnosis, especially when the doctor looked me in the eye and said, "Well, Bob, it happens to be a very rare form of cancer that's incurable." Thank goodness his words never really registered in my brain. I immediately began taking mega-doses of prayer, positive attitude, and productive medicine.

A specialist said to me, "Unless you find a donor somewhere in the world, you'll have less than 18 months." My thought: Who says so? Only the Master Physician knows how long I have! I finally replied, "Where did you come up with that number?" And he said, "I've had 57 patients over seven years who have had the same cancer cell makeup that you have and only one is still living."

He's telling me I have two out of 58 chances? I'll take those odds! Never put a period where God put a comma. Today, I'm cancer free!

—BOB MOAWAD

strongerthancancer

Faith is the substance of things hoped for,
the evidence of things not seen.

**—Hebrews 11:1**

The marriage contract! I remember, saying…"for better, for worse, for richer, for poorer"…but I don't remember, "stem cell transplant" being included. It didn't exist in those days. To newlyweds in their twenties, a long-term illness is merely a remote and distant possibility.

But 30 years later the harsh words and the harsh reality of a multiple myeloma diagnosis to my perfectly healthy husband sent sound waves reverberating through my brain. Fear was my initial reaction. And then somehow, miraculously, the word Faith crept in to calm me. Complete trust in my God overwhelmed me. Bob's fate was in God's hands, and that's the best place it could possibly be. My job was to go along.

Typically, Bob chose to put his "bulldog" teeth into his cancer. And we have had some wonderful things to be thankful for: great family support, good friends, each other and a good sense of humor! Today, 2-1/2 years later, my husband Bob is cancer free.

—ANDREA MOAWAD

11

It will be four years in February since everyone I went to told me there was nothing they could do. But there was one doctor who believed I had a 50-50 chance, and that's all I needed to hear.

—CAROL MAATA

Never give up! Sixteen years ago I was given six months to live. My husband and I fired that doctor and sought a second opinion.

—MARYLOU CRABILL

June, 1995. As I sat on the end of an exam table, I heard the doctor say I only had three to six months to live. With all the strength I could muster, I said to him, "Excuse me, Doctor, but God has created me, and He might have other plans for my life."

Seven years have passed. Many doctors have seen me, many treatments, many labs, many X rays, but God is still in charge and has never stopped working in my life. Your best plan to fight cancer is to set the dire predictions aside and start with friends, family and your Creator on your side.

—PEGGY LOU SMITH

strongerthancancer

Never let your fears hold you back
from pursuing your hopes.
—John F. Kennedy

I was 40 when I was diagnosed with a rare type of colon cancer.  In 1995, they told me I might live 18 months if I did chemo and radiation.  That night I thought, "I won't get to see my girls get married, won't see my only son grow up, never be a grandma."  I told my husband then and there that if I'm only going to live for 18 months I will not die a pauper's death.  We took trips and did a lot of things that we were waiting until we retired to do.

Well, the bad news is that we spent all our retirement funds.  The good news is that I'm here years later enjoying my two new grandchildren.  Although I consider myself a strong person, I believe that God gives life and He takes it.  We think we're running the show but we aren't.  Should this disease someday take my life, I don't want anyone to say that I gave up, lost hope, or refused to try the latest treatment. I want them to remember that God gave me life and He has just taken me home—not when the doctors said I would go, but when He decided I would go.

—TRUDY JANSEN

> You are alive, and that is the only place
> you need to be to start.
>
> **—Carrie Rainey**

When my wife, Betty, was diagnosed with breast cancer, we were both in shock. How could I best help Betty? I immediately went to the Internet and started educating myself. I learned very quickly what to expect and what questions to ask. From that point on, whenever the doctors talked, I knew what they were saying and could help Betty fill in the blanks.

The treatments started and I was with her every step of the way. June 27th was a GREAT day— the last radiation treatment. Betty packed up and left for home.

Our thanks go out to the many doctors and staff, my brother who phoned long distance five times a week to see how we were doing, our parents who helped morally and financially, and our employees who were very understanding at a time of family crisis. Family and friends are a very powerful thing. Don't ever underestimate it. We are living proof that a family who shares everything—the good, the bad, and the ugly—can overcome anything, including cancer.

—ALAN TIPPLE

strongerthancancer

The human spirit is stronger than anything
that can happen to it.
—George C. Scott

I know I wouldn't have survived 5-plus years with my very aggressive cancer had it not been for my husband's spirit and strength. I know my husband's advice would be: Don't leave your brain at the door when going to your first oncologist. Also, follow your own true guide within, your own spirit.

My advice would be: Prayer works! When folks ask what they can do for you and your family, ask them to pray for you. If you do have other needs (a ride, a meal, financial help, etc.), ask openly for those too. By asking, you really offer others a chance to give of themselves.

My motto now is, "Everything happens for a reason." Sometimes you get to see the results of the challenges in your life and sometimes you get to practice strengthening your faith.

Dr. Glen Warner from Bellevue, WA told me early on to look for blessings, even in cancer. Hard to imagine, but I've found that it's true.

—LINDA RYAN

> Go ahead and cry. I'll catch your tears.
> **—J. Russell**

You reach your early sixties. You're thankful and you're counting your blessings. Then you meet a wonderful woman late in life and things get even better. Her name is Z, simply Z. A partner, a friend, a lover. How good can it get?

Then the lump and the bad news. My mate has breast cancer. I see the look of terror in her eyes. There is only comfort in protective embraces. I whisper into her ear, "It's going to be okay, we'll make it, this too will pass." This embrace, this whisper will happen several times a day for close to 10 months. The look of terror in her eyes will change to determination.

Z is my heroine. The surgery, the chemo, the baldness, all dealt with on a "one day at a time" basis. Me wearing her wigs and goofing around with her prosthetic bras to lighten the load. The day-to-day march to wellness. Talk about "Character building class 101"—Z has earned her Ph.D. After completing Camp Hell we can laugh a little, cry a little and count our blessings. My sweet Z, I look into your eyes and do a little slow dance with you in my arms, and I count my blessings. What a blessing to count *your* blessings.

—TRUMAN X. JONES

**strongerthancancer**

When I got the phone call I was devastated: Breast
cancer. Thank God for my wonderful husband,
Truman, I shudder to think how I would have gone
through this without his love and support. He was
my salvation, my strength and my hope.

From the time I was diagnosed I was terrified. After
the tears, my husband held me and we talked. He
gave me the courage to go forward. He continually
complimented my good attitude, and we did not
allow the "poor me" syndrome into our lives. I was
given support from my parents, Lois and Cope, and
my children, Janet and Chris; friends and acquaintan-
ces put me on prayer lists. We changed our diet and
followed all the rules for keeping healthy. At all the
doctors meetings it was very important to have
Truman with me to take notes and to ask questions.

Remember, be positive. After my last chemo in
December of 2001, my dear husband took me to
Mexico for a month to celebrate my recovery. We
didn't stay at a big expensive resort, just being together
was enough. Thank you Truman, I love you. Peace.

—JUDY E. LODGE (Z)

# Concern should drive us into action and not into a depression.

—KAREN HORNEY

I think Joan Baez, the folk singer, originally said it, but I have held onto it through all my treatments: "Action is the antidote for despair."

—SANDY BLAIR

Ten years ago when I learned that I would need to undergo mastectomy surgery and also would not be a candidate for reconstruction, my heart sank. I was only 38 and so depressed, but my husband taught me to look at my operation as "transformation surgery."

He said, "The surgeon's mission is to transform you from a victim into a breast cancer survivor. You will sail way up the survival curve by having this surgery and ridding your body of the source of this disease. You are exchanging your breast for another chance at life and that is a very fair trade."

He was right. I now escort breast cancer patients into the operating room at Johns Hopkins, and I share my husband's words of wisdom and strength with each of them.

—LILLIE SHOCKNEY

> It's okay to get down once in awhile,
> as long as you don't get down on yourself.
> **—B.J. Marshall**

It's okay to have days when you're scared to death, and cry and cry, and it's okay to distance yourself from friends, family and even God. Just remember the next day will be better, your family and friends will help you through everything, and God will never leave your side.

—JEANIE GRAHAM

In 1993 I went for a surgical biopsy, cancer was confirmed and I went immediately to the chemo ward. I freaked out! I wanted to leave, punch something, scream…anything to express my fear and anger at this nightmare! In the next few weeks, I resisted the rounds of chemo with all my might and anger!

Later I went to the mall looking for hats, still angry and anticipating my complete baldness. A beautiful lady named Denise spotted me crying in the hat store. She promptly covered me with her coat so no one could see me cry. She told me that she too had cancer and knew how I felt. Her hair was short and

## strongerthancancer

Lend me your hope for awhile.  A time will come
when I will heal and lend my renewed hope to others.
—Eloise Cole

was just growing back from her last and final round
of chemo.  She told me that I needed to say good-
bye to my anger and disbelief, and to welcome the
chemo instead of fighting it, as it will prolong my life.
She also said that I needed to come to peace with
this and with myself in order to survive.

She then gave me a small purple stone that she had
carried with her throughout her entire cancer and
chemo experience. She told me that it had brought
her great peace and luck and that it was time for her
to pass it on.  I kept that stone with me for the year
and a half that it took to get me through this ordeal.
Denise was both an angel and inspiration to me.
She helped me when I wasn't able to help myself.

And she was right.  Starting that day I embraced my
cancer and the chemo treatments with as much
gusto as I had the negative attitude.  I came through
all of this with flying colors, all because I changed my
attitude and my thinking.  I am grateful that I am still
alive, and I now attribute many positive things in my
life to this cancer ordeal.

—MEL BASSETT

21

> Have faith.  God's care will carry you…
> so you can carry others.
> **—Dr. Robert Schuller**

Sure, cancer is a big "disease," but I've learned that God, family, friends and prayer are so much bigger! (P.S. I'm still here).  Amen.

—MARY JOAN OLSON

When cancer strikes an individual in a family, the lives of everybody within the household are changed. I have been a family friend and caretaker to the Payton family for 17 years.  As you might expect, when Walter was diagnosed, we all rolled up our sleeves and worked together as a team.  We were there day and night with him, spiritually, emotionally, socially and physically—just as Walter would have done for any of us.

To the patient, I urge you to never give up, have a positive attitude, and know that your friends and family are right there with you.  To the caregiver, remain firm and focused in your commitment, and radiate your faith to your loved ones.  Keep steadfast in prayer, and always remember that with God all things are possible.

—LUNA PICART

strongerthancancer

The feeling remains that He
is on the journey too.
—**Teresa of Avilla**

As a cancer patient, so far I have learned:

* Don't wait until rough times to develop your relationship with God, family, and friends.

* It's okay to ask God questions; but not okay to demand answers.

* Cancer respects no one, rich or poor.

* Living isn't always easy; accepting that fact makes it easier.

* It is impossible to live our tomorrows today.

* Faith is for the unknown, not the known.

* No trial comes without lessons and assignments. What I choose to do with them is up to me.

* God is faithful!

* As long as there is breath and God, there is hope!

* We are God's PERSONAL touch to other hurting people.

* One cannot live in or change the past or future. That is why God gives us the present.

—RACHEL L. BAILEY

> Time has healed me, but time has not
> made me forget.
>
> **—Janis Heil**

I was diagnosed with Hodgkin's Disease on Dec. 7, 1998 (my own little "D-Day"). I had just turned 36, had a loving husband, two delightful stepdaughters and two sons in first and second grade. I had family, faith, work and friend support like no other. My doctor is Lance Armstrong's famous Doc, Craig Nichols.

What has cancer meant to me, now that I've been free of the disease nearly three years? Cancer taught me to appreciate the line, "Today is a gift, that's why they call it the present!" I do NOT put things off any longer. I do NOT take my health for granted. I do NOT have plans way out there…we plan to do it now.

Nothing really eloquent here, but cancer gave me invaluable gifts: Encouragement, feeling people's prayers, simplicity, and enjoying people's loving me while I was still alive! I also have an attitude of "Thank you God for this too, and for whatever is in store, because I know all things come together for good." I beat the bugger, and my heart breaks for the many fighters who do not. But let's stick together and we will beat this thing, once and for all. We *can* do it!

—COLLEEN LACTER

strongerthancancer

> Doing your best at this moment puts you in
> the best place for the next moment.
> **—Oprah Winfrey**

"Malignant" is an ugly word scrolling around your brain like a screen saver, but when it's officially stamped on a pathology report in huge type, it's a heart-stopper. With hope, help, courage and love you sneak past this initial terror and start the process of repairing your soul. Get moving please! Call any of the organizations whose mission is to help you: 1-800-ACS-2345 (American Cancer Society) or 1-800-4 CANCER (National Cancer Institute) will help. Ask questions and get answers.

Don't go to appointments alone; always take a second brain and set of ears. Find inspiration! Fight for the doctors you want. Pray. Eight million survivors are out there—find one to talk to. And while you're helping yourself, help someone else; you'll feel better. Be your own healthcare Team Leader and, if you can't, enlist someone who can. Most important, hold, hug, embrace, caress and encourage your self well. Work hard and love each day you have. This is the greatest gift! Are we stronger than cancer? Believe it!

—LINDA ROBINSON

Tell the negative committee that
meets in your head to sit down and shut up.
—**Kathy Kendall**

My Aunt Vera has this quotation from Bernie Siegel rubber-banded to her Bible: Cancer patients teach us that life isn't about "Why me?" but "Try me!"
—LOUIE PARALINE

When we feel that we have been dealt an unfair hand, it is easy for us humans to implore, "Why me?" When I was told that I had breast cancer, frankly my response was, "Why not me?" I saw little rhyme or reason as to whom was chosen for this dubious honor of having cancer. I felt that I deserved to escape no more than anyone else. This mindset may seem a negative one, but I found it to be a type of acceptance, as well as empowerment. It led me quickly to the next level of "Why not me?," which was, "Then why not me for the cure?"
—MARY ANN ARMSTRONG

This little thought is submitted in memory of my wife, Lyndall, who lived eight active years, AFTER being told she had a mean survival time of just three months with lung cancer. Lyndall's philosophy: "Get busy living or you will get busy dying."
—ELMER KUBALL

strongerthancancer

A breast cancer diagnosis 10 years ago left me feeling weak and defeated.  After surgery and radiation, I quit feeling sorry for myself and took control of my life again.  I thought, "I am so blessed with a wonderful husband, six of my own children, two beautiful stepchildren, and fifteen grand-children—I need to live, and I intend to."

First, I changed my mental attitude, starting by forgiving everyone in my life, including myself. Next I changed my physical attitude, learning how to eat and live healthy.

From there, I reached out to others.  Now, ten years later, I sit at the front door of Gilda's Club South Florida every day and welcome cancer survivors and their families.  I see them change from being very fearful to taking control of their lives once again as they and their family and friends participate in support and networking groups.  At this time in my life I have moved all the way from giving up to reaching out and making a difference.

—MARY BURCH

When a loved one is battling cancer, one of the strongest and most reassuring things we can say is, "You are in our prayers." But when my sister, Lydia, went in for her bone marrow transplant, we were temporarily cut off from communicating with her. Still, my family found a simple way to let Lydia know every day that we were all praying for her from afar. We all chipped in and bought a cell phone for her. She was not allowed to accept cell phone calls in her hospital room, but we got permission to set the ringer on "vibrate" and then we called her number every time we said a prayer for her, which was often. She couldn't answer, but the vibration from the phone told her we were near and in prayer, every hour of every day throughout her stay.

—ANNIE AVERY

My mom, a beautiful and vivacious woman, was diagnosed with breast cancer. Three months later, she lost both breasts and all her hair. When I first saw her bald, I was speechless. I could see that she had lost her sunny disposition. I struggled with what to say, how to comfort her. I rehearsed empty

strongerthancancer

Hope is like a helium balloon; it can't soar to
the heavens if you hold it down by the string.
—Lyndsey Boucherly

phrases in my head, like "Don't worry, your hair will grow back soon."

Finally, I just went to her and said, "Look Mom, I see what you're going through and don't know what to say, except I'm so sorry you have to go through this. With or without your hair, we love you and we're with you all the way. Now, let's go shopping for some great hats." And we did.

—JENNIFER PFAHLER

A loving family can make the battle so much easier and lighter. Here is a whimsical little poem I wrote about a month after diagnosis when everything was still "up in the air." May it lighten and buoy your spirits too:

**If, If, When…**
If you are diagnosed,
become diagonal.
If you are prognosed,
become protagonal.
When you are healed,
be helium!

—NANCY MCKAY

I think we're here
for each other.

—CAROL BURNETT

> We rise by lifting others.
> —**Robert Green Ingersoll**

When I think of "Team," it's not the Chicago Bears, Bulls or Cubs. Team is my family—Mom, Brittney and Miss Luna—and all our friends who rallied around us when Dad was sick.

—JARRETT PAYTON

Here is one of the most beautiful and powerful phrases in the English language: *"I'm here for you, no matter what."* Each year cancer invades the lives of more than a million families, but God sends friends to our door to soothe our fears and chase away the darkness. "Connie, I'm here for you when you need me"—this is something I heard quite often after Walter was diagnosed. Spoken softly and sincerely from the heart, those simple words meant the world to me.

Typically, our loved ones are looking for something "big" to do, but little things often mean the most. The smile on a friend's face who just stopped by to say "Hi." The sound of laughter filling a room full of friends or family. Or just some regular conversation and a little gossip to provide a welcome change. These are the little things anyone can do and be a hero.

—CONNIE PAYTON

31

When I learned that I had cancer, I thought it was the end of the world, but it was merely an introduction to a whole new world.  God gives us gifts in unusual ways.  When I needed Him most, He sent me friends who taught me how much others could care, could give love, and could give of themselves.

—MARTIN BERKOFSKY

Friends and loved ones make the difference.  The source of strength that has guided me through 15 years of fighting cancer are these simple words from family and friends: "Hang in there—you are in my prayers."

—BONNIE VOSS

Friends and family have to quickly rally around the person who has cancer.  Everyone here at CTCA is a firm believer in the power of faith, friends, and family.  Time and again I've seen people who have been given three months to live come back for their five year celebration of being cancer free!

—MARGARET SNIDER, CTCA

strongerthancancer

> One of the best things to hold onto in life
> is each other.
>
> **—Audrey Hepburn**

I love this passage from D.H. Lawrence and had it framed for my fishing cabin: "I didn't know, until I was at odds with the world, how much my friends who believe in me…mean to me."

—JERRY MALINOWSKY

During my two battles with cancer, I learned that my mother felt every pain, and that she suffered and fought right along with me. Her conviction was, "This too shall pass," and it did!

I learned from my sister that her unconditional love could carry me through the treatment and that we could both be better people for it. She is and always will be my biggest hero.

I learned from my friends that if someone cares for you, the physical scars are of no concern to them.

Finally, I learned that cancer is a coward, it doesn't fight fair and that I must be ever-vigilant against its return.

—KAREN CARTER

Tips For Friends of Cancer Patients:

- Day of surgery—only go if you were personally invited to wait with the family; too many people is overwhelming.

- Bring the family small portions of healthy treats. Oftentimes the family doesn't want to leave the hospital because they are waiting for news to come and they don't eat well.

- Offer to "keep watch" while the family takes a nap.  Let them know you will wake them if a doc comes by.

- A friend made a special pillowcase that was soft, and the fabric was beautiful and meaningful.

- Think comfort: soft pajamas, t-shirts, slippers, linen spray, favorite pillow, blanket, lotion, mints, soft face cloth.

- A friend brought his favorite CD's.  Bring the latest videos—the hospitals have a limited selection.

strongerthancancer

- A medium size pad of paper/pen or a tape recorder to catch doctor's or nurse's notes when there is a lot going on.

- Bring your love—but especially bring smiles and laughter, it gives hope.

- Lots of short visits at the hospital and at home. If it's during the holidays, help with holiday traditions. Put up their tree, bring Easter eggs decorated, etc.

- Home Meals! I initially said no, but thankfully our friends insisted on bringing meals to our house anyway. Those first two weeks back from the hospital are rough and those meals were a welcome sight.

- Short visits! Take the family's lead; sometimes they are exhausted but polite, and feel the need to "host."

- Continue to ask how their progress is going; families with cancer appreciate the care.

- Pray. It works!

—JAN CAPINEGRO

Right after my husband, Jeff, was diagnosed with brain cancer, we were lying in bed thinking about our 7-year-old son, Zach. We made a decision then and there. Although our son would not have a long life with his father, he would witness strength, compassion, honesty and dignity.

We worked to make as many indelible memories as possible. We flew over the Grand Canyon and rode horses through the Arizona desert. Each night I would give our son a medical update. I always asked if he had questions, including the big one, "Is Dad going to die?" I explained that we may not have Dad in our lives as long as other dads, but we would make the most of every second we did have.

One friend volunteered to schedule lunches and dinner out for Jeff with clients and friends who wanted special time with him. Jeff truly looked forward to each meeting and gave a lasting memory of vibrancy and courage. Years later Zach and I still speak openly and lovingly about Jeff every day, and those around us always join in. There is no guarantee how long we have together, but the number of quality

strongerthancancer

You remain my father, philosopher,
counselor, and friend.
—A Son's Prayer

moments and memories we generate is not cancer's
decision, it's truly ours.

—JENNIFER HURWITZ

I was only nine, but I wanted to help. Dad had a
favorite spot on our porch where he'd recuperate,
and that gave me an idea. His forty-fifth birthday
was approaching, so Mom and I went in search of
a present—the fluffiest, most comfortable pillow we
could find. With a black Sharpie marker I carefully
penned the words, "The best Dad in the world" above
the oversized heart upon which his head would rest.

From then on, my dad took his pillow wherever he
went, to the hospital, the MRI office, even to hospice
for his last days with my mom and me.

After Dad's first seizure, the doctors gave him six
months to live, but Dad hung on and we had lots
of time together. Two and a half years after his
diagnosis, through all the love, laughter, and tears, he
fell asleep—on that same pillow—and passed away.
His head still rests on that same spot, right above
"The best Dad in the world."

—ZACH HURWITZ, 16

Our son, John, was six when I was diagnosed with breast cancer. Although we were nervous, we openly shared details of my treatment with him—just the basics, using simple words—and we highly recommend it.

For example, we described chemo as "superhero medicine, strong enough to knock the hair right off my head," and John got excited about my baldness instead of shocked. When we explained about the upcoming mastectomy, he concocted his own creative ways for the doctor to get the sickness out while leaving my breast intact (Don't ask; one involved using a spoon!). And so he had time to get used to the idea.

We stayed close to each other the entire way. I actually put John to bed every night of the 21 days I spent in the bone marrow transplant unit—over the phone! He "read" picture books to me while I rested during radiation. By including our son in my healing process, we empowered him—and made me feel a lot better too.

—LORI MISICKA

strongerthancancer

> Laughter is an essential amino acid.
> —Patch Adams

As I went through my own battle with breast cancer—thankfully now in remission—the hardest thing was how to tell my teenage children. They remembered how their grandmother lost her battle with cancer. My husband and I told them together and simply stressed that while no one could predict the future, I was going to do everything in my power to get well, and whatever happened, and whether I was sick or well, their dad and I would always be there for them. We then did our best to live a normal family life, neither sugarcoating reality nor dwelling on the most awful possibilities.

Humor was so important. My kids liked it when I draped my wig (nicknamed "Muskrat Susie" for its gray-brown color) on a broomstick and danced with it in the family room. One day, while I was at treatment, my daughter lightened one of my darkest moments by painting elaborate makeup on the face of my wig form. Then she set it in my room, where a luxurious bath by candlelight had been thoughtfully arranged, with this note: "Remember, Mom, you ARE beautiful!"

—PATRICIA ARTIMOVICH

In 1998, my husband was diagnosed with pancreatic cancer. My advice to every family is to look cancer right in the eye. Discuss what the ill person's wishes and hopes are for the children. These talks can be painful, but they cheat cancer of any victory over your spirit, and will be comforting in the future.

—GINGER SWIERENGA

To all the children reading this book: I was only 14 when I lost my father. He was truly more than a father to me, he was my friend, my hero, and I was in every sense of the word a daddy's girl. His passing was such a crisis for me. For awhile I didn't think that I would survive his death. If you are going through that kind of pain, please don't withdraw; instead, reach out to those who love you.

With the help of a counselor, my family and my faith I began to realize that my world had not come to an end. In a very real way even my relationship with my father has not ended. You see, I learned many things from Dad and will carry them forever in my heart. I remember a place called hope. I remember how my father, in his short time on earth, touched so many

strongerthancancer

> To live in the hearts we leave behind is not to die.
> **—Thomas Campbell**

lives—how he took the time to make all those who crossed his path feel special.

Last but not least, I learned that change of any type requires courage, the kind of courage my father inspired in others. Today our family continues to fight cancer, and we will until the day a cure is found. That's the way he would have wanted it.

—BRITTNEY PAYTON

Throughout Walter's battle with cancer, he would occasionally do something that would later become very important to the children. Every now and then one of the kids would complain to me that, "Dad has taken over my room." I'd go take a look and, sure enough, Walter would be sleeping in Jarrett's bed or watching TV in Brittany's room.

I think Walter knew exactly what he was doing because, after he passed, the kids were elated that he had spent so much time in their rooms. They really felt his presence, his strength and peacefulness in their hearts.

—CONNIE PAYTON

When my father, a proud man, was diagnosed with colon cancer, he became depressed. His oncologist assured us that his cancer was very treatable, but Dad had pretty much given up hope. The adults in our family tried to rally his spirits but nothing worked.

One day, my 9-year-old daughter, Katrina, showed up with a little wooden box for her Papa. Katrina had painted a bear on the lid that looked just like Dad, and next to the bear were two words: *Papa's Worries.* Katrina instructed Dad to write down his worries every night on a little piece of paper and put them in the worry box. "When you wake up, Papa," she promised, "all your worries will be smaller."

For the first time in weeks I saw my dad's eyes light up. He not only rallied and fought—he won! Today, years later, Dad will be the first to tell you that Katrina's little box is his most treasured possession.

—ROGER FLYNN

Tell people that kids want to help, we need to help, we really can help—please let us help.

—FRED PEREZ, 11

strongerthancancer

> I don't look at what I've lost.
> I look instead at what I have left.
> **—Betty Ford**

The day after my double mastectomy, my 9-year-old daughter came to see me. She put her face very close to me and I said, "What are you looking at?" She said, "Well Mum, you are still beautiful inside and I can see it shining out." That still makes me cry.

The day after I was diagnosed we were in the bank and they were selling little yellow flowers to pin on and she wanted one. After I bought it for her, she asked, "Why does it have cancer care written on it?" I said it is because the money we pay goes to cancer care. "Oh well," she laughed, "you will certainly get your money's worth, won't you!" She has been wonderful right from the start and I am very lucky to have her.

—MISHCA

At 33, when I was diagnosed with breast cancer, my 16-year-old son gave me this quote: "Never knock on Death's door. Ring the doorbell and run. Death hates that!"

—MICHELLE WHEELER

He was my best friend and business partner, so Bob's cancer diagnosis sent me into shock. Devastating news about someone you've admired, loved and worked with for over a quarter of a century will do that. I felt helpless, and every day I prayed to determine what might help and encourage him most.

Then, I saw people spring into action! Our office staff daily doing projects to keep things going. Family and friends starting prayer chains in their respective churches. A torrent of cards, letters and e-mails providing support and encouragement from all over. Everyone's awareness growing, everyone's love expanding, everyone supporting in his or her own way. The result? Thanks to medical advancements, abounding support, God's grace, and my friend's indomitable spirit, his health has been restored!

—DICK ANDERSON

I love this, it was on the wall at St Anthony's Health Center: "Don't avoid me just because I'm ill. Be the friend, the loved one, you've always been. Weep with me when I weep. Laugh with me when I laugh. Don't be afraid to share this with me. Call me first, but

strongerthancancer

don't be afraid to visit.  I need you, I get lonely.
Bring me a positive attitude—it's catching!  Help
me celebrate today, tomorrow—life!"

—ESTELLE CAPUTO

We lost a great warrior when we lost Walter Payton,
but in many ways he is still with us and will *always* be
with us.  Walter raised national awareness about
organ donation and showed the world how to fight
with dignity.  His great hope was that the fight would
continue through each and every one of us until we
finally knock it out and find a cure.

Part of his legacy is that now we as a nation can put
a hero's face to a disease that many of us believed
couldn't touch us.  I know it has truly changed the
way that I look at cancer, because I always thought it
only happened to people who don't take care of
themselves.  Now Walter's family is carrying the torch
to eliminate this monster once and for all.  We must
team up with the Payton Family, and with all other
cancer-fighting organizations, in a combined battle to
find a cure to this deadly disease, once and for all.

—THOMAS SANDERS,
  *FRIEND AND FORMER TEAMMATE.*

The world knows
very little of its
greatest heroes.

—DON WARD

> Some of the best and bravest people
> will never be featured on the ten o'clock news.
> —Dan Zadra

Something we need to teach our children: not all heroes are honored in a big parade. There are everyday people all across the country who are quietly battling cancer and whose courage would easily eclipse the caped crusaders.

—TERRI ATKINSON
*HOSPICE*

I just celebrated 12 years of remission from severe aplastic anemia. I often tell my husband, Ben, that he is one of the greatest heroes in my life because I was given this path to walk, but he *chose* it right beside me.

—TIFFANY LOREN ROWE

I watched as you raised our family, and I watched as you, who are so small, stared down cancer. You have been my light, my friend, my mother—then and now—and more than that, my hero.

—PAT COVINA
*A LETTER TO HOME*

"**Y**our son has a brain tumor." The words still resonate in my mind. Here sat this handsome and otherwise healthy man who was 37 and the father of five small children. I watched as the doctors told him to go home and get his life in order. His response was so typical of my son: "That is not acceptable."

Throughout his treatment he has refused to let his condition take over his life. One day after his first operation I saw him walk from the recovery room on his own two feet. He has returned to running 5-K Runs, usually for cancer events. He knows that his family, friends and Medical Team are behind him, and that seems to give him unlimited strength. Whenever we travel to see his doctors, his first remark is, "It could always be worse and there are people much more ill than me."

There are others like my son. They are the everyday people who refuse to be beaten down by cancer. They are not famous, and very few people know their names. But here's my name for them: *Hero.*

—EDWARD D. FLANIGAN SR.

strongerthancancer

I am eleven and have a program called "Heavenly Hats" for cancer patients. So far I have delivered more than 5,000 hats to about 50 different hospitals. I have also been able to visit with a lot of cancer patients. All of them usually talk to me about how happy they are that I started this program, because being able to receive a brand-new hat in the hospital means so much to them.

Many have told me how hard it is to look so different without hair. It seems like the younger boys and girls really have a hard time with this. To be able to see the smile on their face when I give them a new hat made all the hard work for this program worthwhile. Most of the people seem so brave, they are heroes to me, but I know they are all scared too. I tell them not to worry, that everyone is pulling for them, and that my grandma, who had cancer, has been cancer-free for five years now.

Hats off to everyone who is fighting cancer!
—ANTHONY LEANNA

Walter was a hero both on and off the field. He never lost his sense of humor and he never complained. He focused on us as a family and he never said, "Why me?" Walter always seemed more concerned about everybody else. He wanted us to know how important we all were to him, and in turn, we wanted him to know how much he meant to us.

The many wonderful things he did for so many people were never made known because that's the way Walter wanted it. He relished the fact that he could bring happiness to so many people. For him, that meant everything. Nothing more needed to be said.

—CONNIE PAYTON

If you ask me how I want to be remembered, it is as a winner. You know what a winner is? A winner is somebody who has given his best effort, who has tried the hardest they possibly can, who has utilized every ounce of energy and strength within them to accomplish something.

It doesn't mean that they accomplished it or failed, it means that they've given it their best. That's a winner.

—WALTER PAYTON

strongerthancancer

If children with cancer can find hope, joy, and
courage in their day—and they do—why can't we?
—DAN ZADRA

I was diagnosed when I was 13 and am now 23.
To the parents of a child fighting cancer, I would say,
"Keep your child thinking, but not about how ill they
feel. Keep them active…put up a mini basketball
hoop in their room, play Nintendo. Most importantly,
always be there for them. Knowing that someone is
there to go through it with you…it's so comforting.

To the young patients, remember this card was dealt
to us. We gotta step up to the challenge, we have no
choice. This helps define who we are. Have strength
and courage and know that sometimes you have to
feel worse before you can feel better, but after you've
finally come through your treatment, take it from me:
you'll know from that day forward that you can
overcome anything!
—TAMI NELSON

When my son, Tony, was diagnosed at 15 with a rare familial cancer, it was the support of faith, family, and friends that literally carried us.

Our good friend Father Jim, a Catholic priest, came over to bless Tony before he had brain and spinal surgery. Father asked Tony if he thought he may have done something to deserve cancer—and to my shock, Tony said yes. Father quickly explained that our God is a God of love, not a punishing God. That during this time Tony would see God's love shine through others.

And did it ever! Every prayer, card, visit, balloon, flower, cookie, CD, message, book, treat, etc., sustained us all. Don't worry about doing the "right thing" for the family—do anything, do something.

Our parish friends and family also went to mass on the day of the surgery. Knowing that there were almost 200 people (mostly teens!) in church and praying filled our hearts with hope and strength.

—JAN CAPINEGRO

strongerthancancer

Alone we can do so little.
Together we can do so much.
—**Helen Keller**

My sister, Betsy, was thirteen when she was diagnosed with Hodgkin's disease, and her first request was to have her sisters at home with her. I was a college senior at the time, attending Northwestern University. My sister Katey, then 20, was attending college closer to home. I borrowed a friend's car for the weekend and drove the four hours back to my hometown, Grand Rapids, Michigan.

Katey and I spent the weekend watching movies with Betsy, playing games and laughing about how Betsy was going to beat her cancer. My parents used Katey and me as sounding boards for their concerns about Betsy's condition. We listened as they explained how helpless they felt and how they hoped the insurance company would cover everything. About seven months after her diagnosis, Betsy was in remission. She was and is "stronger than cancer" and remains an inspiration to everyone who knows her. I and countless others who know and love Betsy were not able to do anything specific to help her heal, but sometimes just being there is enough.

—EMILY BREUKER

> Attitudes are more important than facts.
> **—Dr. Karl Menninger**

Every family is like a garden.  Each friend or loved one is like a flower in that garden.  They each have their own beauty and their own special spot in the soil.  When cancer touches a loved one, ask yourself, "What is my role, my special spot?"

—CAROLYN JETT

A strange thing happened on the way to helping my brother with a bone marrow procedure.  I had my twelve tubes of blood sent to Fred Hutchinson Cancer Center in Seattle and the next day, "Pow," the report came back that I had CLL.  I was flabbergasted to say the least.  All I was trying to do was save my brother and then this most disturbing diagnosis.

Even though I couldn't be there with my blood for my brother, I know we are both here for each other.  Already he is experiencing a positive turnaround, is cancer free, and is inspiring me in my battle.  It's no surprise that a strong faith, supportive family, and a positive will to survive are what makes us stronger than cancer.

—JOHN F. MOAWAD

strongerthancancer

The phone rang as I sat on my bed.  Like a bad
dream, I heard my mom saying, "Your dad has
cancer."  I was stunned, shocked and scared.
I asked, "What kind of cancer?" and she responded,
"Multiple myeloma.  It's not a 'good' one to get, if
there is such a thing."

As I hung up the phone, I laid down on my bed and
began to cry.  You see, when your dad is your hero
and role model, and you are his namesake, you never
imagine this could happen.  I began to get angry;
then I went to the computer to research multiple
myeloma and became even more depressed.

I thought, "This cancer wants to take my dad away
from me!"

But my dad had other plans.  It has not been easy,
but today, two and a half years later, my hero has
weathered his treatments and is now cancer-free.
He is, we are, and you are stronger than cancer.

—BOB MOAWAD, JR.

55

Twenty years ago I lost one of my best friends to cancer when we were only sixteen. I used to curse God for allowing leukemia to take Todd's life. I watched as the cancer grew and Todd slowly disappeared. I used to wonder how someone could go from 135 pounds to a mere 48 and still remain so strong and upbeat. I didn't realize then that cancer may take our body, but it can't touch our spirit.

Last year I got married. Todd's mom was there and I hadn't seen her in years, yet it felt as if he and I had just come in from playing outdoors. Her hugs still felt the same, and I know my old buddy was there with me, just as he has been every day along the way.

I often thank Todd for this strange perspective I developed. I was a soccer player growing up and continue an active lifestyle today. There was peer pressure then, just as there is for any kid today, but Todd gave me the strength to say no. I remember sitting in the hospital with him and then seeing our friends at a party later that evening. I used to stand by and watch them fritter away life by drinking, smoking or doing drugs. I'd watch them play with

Some of the most important
things in life aren't things.
**—Linda Ellerbee**

the greatest gift of all—their health—and think about
my buddy lying in his hospital bed.  What a shame.

Cancer may have shortened Todd's life, but it
couldn't touch his spirit.  He's the reason life is so
special to me today.  He's the reason I don't drink,
the reason I try to look for the good in every kid, the
reason I give people another chance.  He's the reason
I know we are stronger than cancer.

—TOTE YAMADA

If there's a silver lining, it's this:  You never realize
how many people you've touched until something like
cancer comes into your life.  It's unbelievable—the
e-mails, cards, letters, calls.  Some of them make me
smile, and some make me cry.  I have had e-mails
from players I coached years ago who say, "I'll never
forget the day when…" and you think, "Wow, I never
realized it meant that much."  That kind of love from
even one person gives you strength for yourself and
strength for the battle.

—CLIVE CHARLES,
  UNIVERSITY OF PORTLAND SOCCER COACH

# Grace under pressure.

—ERNEST HEMINGWAY

> We have loved the stars too fondly
> to be fearful of the night.
> **—John and Phoebe Brashear**

Hospice patients often teach us how to live and love life, despite our own mortality. A patient gave me this thought from Victor Hugo, a treasure: "In the midst of winter I finally learned that within me lies an invincible summer."

—KYLE SHIPLEY
*HOSPICE*

My family witnessed first-hand one September evening that love will out-last and out-shine anything that cancer can do. My grandparents had a wonderful marriage. They used to square dance. When my grandfather was diagnosed with a fatal blood cancer, he lived more than nine months because of the love of my grandmother. He wanted to celebrate her 80th birthday with her.

On the night of her birthday they began to dance. It was as if they were in another place and time. That night my grandfather glided like the gentleman we knew him to be and swept her off her feet. A lifetime of open, honest love was reflected in the power and beauty of that magical evening. No, not even cancer could disturb what they shared.

—ELIZABETH SABO

When my grandmother was diagnosed with cancer I didn't know what to say or how to help. I was just a teenager with nothing to contribute. I was afraid to ask questions, and even more afraid of the answers.

My family decided it would be good for all 10 grandchildren to each sign up for a different weekend to help Grandma out. On my day, she was elated to see me. She had already made one of her ham and cheese sandwiches and put some personal things of hers aside as gifts for me.

We went to work in her garden; Grandma wouldn't let me do it alone. We had such a good time that day, just weeding and talking. For the longest time I forgot all about her cancer, and I think she did too. I realized then that my grandma was still the same person—a lot stronger and a little sadder—but still the same person I'd known and loved all my life. What grace!

I also learned that I had something to contribute; I wasn't helpless after all. Just being there for Grandma was everything to her. And helping my grandma in her garden was one of the best gifts *I've* ever received and has left me with memories I'll treasure forever.

—CONNIE McMARTIN

strongerthancancer

I'll never forget how my grandmother's smile lit up the room every time my brother Mike and I would visit. When she survived a triple bypass heart surgery, she laughed because she could bend over and tie her shoes without effort for the first time in years. She never learned to drive and worked as a cook in a Seattle hospital until she became ill again with breast cancer.

Her courage was such an inspiration to me. I remember going to visit her house as a small child and being sad that she was sick. She had a beautiful weeping willow tree in her front yard that reached to the sky and then touched the ground. I said, "Grandma, why is that tree so sad?" She told me that the tree wasn't really weeping, it only bent down when Mike and I were there so that it could be closer to us!

I will never forget her words of wisdom, humor and comfort as she fought so hard to bring joy to her family in what should have been her own time of need. Courage? My grandmother showed cancer a thing or two.

—DEBBIE OSBORN

My mom took care of Grandma when she was diagnosed with colon cancer. I was 2000 miles away from someone who meant the world to me, and planning my wedding. I was praying that Gram would be able to come, but knowing she probably couldn't.

On a trip home my mom and Grandma were cleaning out the attic. Grandma was a "saver." There, in an old trunk, she came across her wedding dress from fifty years ago. I tried it on so Grandma could see me as a bride, and it fit! Mom took it to the cleaners, had the lace replaced with antique lace from a flea market, and I had the most beautiful dress ever. It was exactly what I would have picked out!

Gram didn't make it to my wedding, but she was wrapped around me all day long. She died eight days later. I learned that sometimes the tasks that you most dread can be the ones that bring such joy. I will always be grateful for Mom deciding to clean out the attic and doing it with Gram…a great memory in a difficult time. Make good memories whenever you can, they are always and forever stronger than cancer.

—KRISTIN WOLFF GASSNER

strongerthancancer

The day before my surgery for breast cancer was very difficult, needless to say. I had to check into the hospital a day early for additional tests and had been in and out of my room all day.

That night I still didn't know whether a lumpectomy or a total mastectomy would be done—that decision would be made by the surgeon while I was on the table. As the day drew to a close, my husband Rick and I tried to pass the night as pleasantly as possible.

When he left, I don't think I've ever felt so alone. I went into the bathroom, and there, on the mirror was the sweetest card. As I opened my suitcase— another card—this man had been busy during my trips in and out of the room. When I got my book to read before bed—another card.

How silly I had been. Yes, I was in an empty room, but I certainly wasn't alone. Thank you, Honey, those cards brought me love and assurance that, no matter what, it would turn out okay—and it did.

—VICKIE GIRARD

I remember the day I told my six-year-old daughter, Hope, that her grandfather had advanced cancer. She asked me if Grandpa was going to die. I told her that everyone dies sooner or later, and that since Grandpa was in his seventies, he couldn't be with us a whole lot longer, even if he beat the cancer. I then told her that while it was so very sad and scary for Grandpa to be so sick, it was also a great gift we'd been given, to have a chance to say all the things to him we want to say. How much we love him, how much he meant to our lives, and that we would never forget him.

Hope and I then talked about how every time we're with someone we love, we never know if it's the last time we'll ever be with that person. It makes it so important for us to tell and show our love, and to treasure the time we have together. It's been over a year since Dad died. Hope tells me that at night she asks him to guide her, just as I have continued to do with my grandfather.

—SHERI ZIEMANN

strongerthancancer

> This is not the end, we'll meet again. God's promise
> will be kept. But all the same, I feel no shame in all
> the tears I've wept.
> **—Forest R. Whatley**

When news broke of Walter's illness, he was always honest and straightforward. When asked by the press, "Are you scared?" he quickly responded, "Hell yes, I'm scared. Keep me in your prayers." How odd to hear what sounded like a plea from someone who always appeared to be so stout and fearless. But courage isn't the absence of fear, it's the affirmation of faith and life *despite* the fear.

There is no such thing as faith without doubt. Walter and I shared our faith in God, and it helped us both deal with our fears and doubts. The power of prayer guided us through a stage in our lives that was not planned or welcomed, but together we faced what fate had dealt us. We trusted with all our heart the promise in the bible, "With God, all things are possible."

Walter eventually died, and I survived. No question, this is very difficult, but I know Walter's message to you would be a message of hope: Do not lose faith, do not despair. Life goes on, it must go on. In fact, it is by living out our lives with the memories of our loved ones sheltered safely in our hearts, that we honor and cherish them best.

—CONNIE PAYTON

I am a single mother, 37, raising three children alone. We have been fighting ovarian cancer in my 15-year-old daughter, Heather, since April 16, 2002. Now, I ask you, how can there be blessings in this? But believe me, there are.

First, we are young and have an uncommon type of tumor, so Heather and I are hoping that our treatment will be successful and that this will help doctors to treat young females like her in the future. Heather wants you to know that if we're all in this battle together, she's doing her part.

What other blessings do we have? We believe in God, we have our faith!!! We are being treated at one of the best cancer treatment facilities in the United States. We have wonderful family and friends, and my daughter has a loving boyfriend who has been by her side through all of this. He is an angel. And I have rekindled a lost friendship with an old best friend, and she is now back in my life.

Another blessing: Since May, Heather has been a Make-A-Wish child and is waiting for her wish to

**strongerthancancer**

meet Nelly and the St. Lunatics, and we heard on July 8th that they have put us on the top of the list to meet them. She is so excited! So you see, good things do come to those who wait. Good things come from cancer as well, but not on their own—we have to fight for them, and Heather and I intend to.

This experience is new, but already it has changed us forever. I would not wish the experience on anyone, but the other side is that my family has a totally different outlook on life now.

Live each day to the fullest because you never know when it will be taken away from you. Never ever take friends or family for granted. I love my daughter, and I love my family, and if our experiences can help someone else in life, then great. Let's be stronger than cancer. Together we can. We intend to continue on until we are cancer-free.

—DORA J. MARTINEZ

I am not a victim.
I am a survivor.

—LANCE ARMSTRONG

Take charge of your thoughts.
Get started…and keep going.
**—Diane Roger**

My head was spinning, trying to process the news.  My breast cancer had metastasized to the surrounding tissue.  A new doctor walked into the exam room and gave me the most amazing advice:

"You were surprised it came back because you thought it was gone.  From now on here's what I recommend.  You get the very best conventional medicine, and we have very good doctors here.  Then you also do alternative medicine (nutrition, supplements, etc).  Then there is your faith, and prayer, and your calling as a pastor.  You keep your eyes fixed on what God has called you to do, and don't think like a victim.  You take care of the cancer like you would the dirty dishes.  You don't let it consume your life or it has already won."

I was numb with shock, and so he did not think I would remember anything of what he said.  But his straight talk was a blessing for me, and I hope it will be a blessing for all.

**—PASTOR LOUISE STOUB**

69

> We define ourselves by the best that is in us,
> not the worst that has been done to us.
> **—Edward Lewis**

We may be diagnosed with cancer, but we are NOT cancer. We can still love, laugh, give, receive, forgive, be grateful, have a sense of humor—in other words, live fully, even with physical limitations.

My life has been greatly enriched by fellow cancer patients. We have shared stories, hopes, dreams, tears, disappointments and losses, humor and helpful suggestions. It has been a journey I would not have chosen, but God—because He is good—has always been present to love me, meet my every need and use it all for His greater good.

—CORA BEHRENS

When someone is diagnosed with cancer, it is important for them to remember that they are not the disease. Our patients here are known by their first names, not their room numbers. When patients come here, it's like coming to an extended family. My grandfather was treated here, and I try to treat every patient with the same love, respect and honor that I would expect for my own grandfather or any other

strongerthancancer

Instead of wallowing, I just made some changes.
—**Stephanie Mills**

loved one.  When it comes to cancer, we are all in this
together, and together we are always stronger.
—ANDREA GILBERTSON, CTCA

After hearing the words, "You have colon cancer"
in April, 2000, I decided to view my illness not as a
potential death sentence but as an opportunity for
growth.  All through my surgery, chemotherapy and
radiation, I lived my plan—to discover what I wanted
in my life and to encourage others living with cancer
to focus on the positive.

During difficult times I also relied on my Buddhist
practice, including relaxation, chanting and
meditation.  My plan included working with the Colon
Cancer Alliance where I learned that knowledge,
understanding and hope can take the place of fear.

Today I am healthier than ever!  I follow a medically
supervised integrated approach to maintaining good
nutrition and health.  Remember: You are not your
tumor.  You are a vital, living individual.  Make your
plan and live!
—DEBORAH KANTER

> Laughter in the face of reality is probably
> the finest sound there is.
> **—Linda Ellerbee**

We were so glad to have my husband, Steve, home from the hospital. He had been diagnosed with acute lymphocytic leukemia three weeks earlier and was taking a high dose of Prednisone to counter the effects of the chemo. Steve likes to landscape. The lush hedge in front of our home was about three-feet high, so he decided to trim it. Later, he called me to take a look—and I gasped. What greeted me was a pathetic row of 12-inch sticks!

Trying not to upset Mr. Prednisone, I asked him gently what had happened. He smiled sheepishly, "Well, they kept looking uneven!" It took weeks for the leaves to grow back, and every day we chuckled, thinking about what our neighbors must have been saying. "Look! There's the chemo house! Even their bushes are on chemo." And they sure looked like it!

Every summer, now, I smile when Steve pulls out the shears. I remember when finding the humor in anything helped us make it through the most challenging time of our lives. Two key learnings: 1) He who laughs, lasts. 2) Never give a man on Prednisone electric shears."

**—KAREN TALKEN**

strongerthancancer

One hot summer morning I received confirmation of breast cancer. To my rescue came my wonderful husband, Marshall, and dear friends. After my treatments, Marshall took me out to purchase 250 daffodil and tulip bulbs. Surely, having something special to look forward to (the expectation of a new flower garden, new life) would help win the battle— and it did!

My diagnosis was in 1987 and now, 15 years later, at age 78, I have found new meaning to my life through my work with the American Cancer Society, and through Random Acts of Kindness, helping to spread joy and service through my community. There really is life after cancer and we really are stronger!

P.S. I lost my dear Marshall not too long ago. But, to this day, whenever I see a patch of daffodils, I am reminded that if we just stick together in faith and hope, we can and will defeat this disease!

—BETTY KIELER

> The dictionary has a lot of "C" words. They include Compassion, Curiosity, Courage and Cuddles.
> —Linda Scott

I received the news of breast cancer one afternoon while at work. I don't recall much after the radiologist announced the big "C" word. I don't even remember driving home. My mother died in 1969 from liver cancer; my mind kept telling me I would die like my mother.

Fortunately there is more than one big "C" word. Christ is a C word, and so is Cancer Treatment Centers of America. About two weeks after diagnosis, I located and dialed their 800-number. Explaining my situation to a kind female voice, I was told someone would call me. Within the hour, I was contacted, and I have never looked back!

Faith in myself, faith in CTCA Tulsa, faith in God, and the support and love of family continue to sustain me. Are we stronger than cancer? My answer is simple: We are!

—LELIA "LEE" BREAUX OLIVIER

strongerthancancer

> A great pleasure in life is doing
> what people say cannot be done.
> **—Walter Bagehot**

It has been a little over five years since I was told I had only a "few months" to live.  Typically, only one percent of liver cancer patients survive, but I have been cancer free for 16 months.  Here's what I've learned from this experience:

First, never lose faith.  God is the Greatest Physician, and whenever we are given a life sentence, it is merely the opinion of man and not the word of God.

Second, look at the word "cancer."  The first three letters spell CAN.  It may sound corny, but with friends, family, good physicians and, oh yes, God by our side, we really CAN take control of cancer and not let it take control of us.

—FAY ANN POLSON

A little prayer that I often said during recovery, and is still a comfort to me:  *God, You're going to be up all night.  You can worry about it.  I need to get some sleep.*

—MARY AUGUSTINE

75

Each of us has a
spark of life inside us,
and we must set off
that spark in one
another.

—KENNY ANSUBEL

> I discovered I always have choices,
> and one of them is a choice of attitude.
> **—Judith Knowlton**

Faith in God and family is what carried me through the dark days and nights when I was diagnosed with lung cancer in July 2001. I believe that God is the one who sent me to a team of physicians who believe in treating the whole person—mind, body and spirit. I now have a different attitude. I realize that cancer is not a death sentence, but only a disease which will have to continually be monitored. My daughter, Lisa, has a quote on her refrigerator that sums up my insight on this battle: "Any fact facing us is not as important as our attitude toward it, for that determines our success or failure."

—BRADY CARINESS

Everyone uses the phrase, "attitude is everything," but I think cancer fighters are the ones who know what it really means. My husband cried when he was diagnosed with terminal cancer at age 35. Then he looked at me and said, "I will beat this!" and never cried again. His indomitable spirit and attitude gave him and us many years longer than anyone ever dreamed.

—LINDA SEVON

Always look forward with high expectations of a full and meaningful life.  Here is a wonderful affirmation that we have shared on our survivor's website and in our support groups: *I shall pass through this world but twice—once before cancer and once after cancer. Let the "after" be the most treasured.*

—CHERYL CALECA,
*LINK TO LIFE NEWSLETTER*

In May 1996, our two little daughters, Sara and Laura, jumped for joy as we brought their new baby brother, Luke, home from the hospital.

Five weeks later my 35 year-old husband, Steve, was diagnosed with an acute leukemia rarely found in adults.  We were shocked and overwhelmed.  How could a perfectly healthy man who exercises regularly and doesn't smoke or drink—how could he possibly be stricken with such a life-threatening illness?

Steve's oncologist concluded that he needed a stem cell transplant from a donor.  Steve had only one sibling, his brother John, who was tested to be a

What, at first, appears to be the end of the road
may merely be a bend in the road.
—Dr. Robert Schuller

donor.  Knowing that the odds of a perfect match
were only twenty percent, we said, "This one's yours,
Lord!"  John turned out to be a perfect match!

On the big day, I began documenting our family's
real-time miracle.  I videotaped the process of
harvesting the life-saving cells, a gift from one brother
to another.  Then I videotaped the transplant process
at St. Luke's hospital.  In 1996, the process was so
new that Steve was the hospital's very first allogeneic
transplant. (Notice the interesting coincidence: Baby
Luke; Leukemia; St. Luke's Hospital.)

October 31,1996 was Steve's new birthday, so we
celebrated accordingly.  We brought in cake,
banners, and balloons and sang "Happy Birthday"
to him as the new stem cells entered his catheter.  It's
the best birthday party ever! Today Steve has made
a complete recovery and our family has rejoiced
every day.  Throughout the cancer experience, we
chose to "never put a period where God had placed
a comma!"

—KAREN TALKEN

How do you know it's bad?  At the age of 79, my father
was diagnosed with bladder cancer.  That sounds
pretty bad, but it turned out to be good.  You see, an
operation successfully removed the cancer but also
disclosed an unrelated, pre-existing condition—fluid
on the brain.  The doctors immediately repaired this
problem too.

Later they told him, "If you had not had the operation
for cancer, we wouldn't have discovered the fluid
problem and you would have soon died from pressure
on the brain."  Dad is now 81 with a clean bill of health,
no cancer and a healthy brain.  He loves to tell people,
"Thank God for cancer.  It saved my life."

—DENNIS GOIN

Cancer is like a blind date that you don't really want to
go on.  After it is all over, it really wasn't as bad as you
thought it was. . . but it certainly wasn't as good as it
could have been. . .and you're definitely not interested
in continuing the relationship.  Take each day as it
comes, pull together with family and friends, and don't
worry about anything that hasn't happened yet.

—ROXANNE ATKINS

strongerthancancer

How beautiful it is to be able to say to someone, "I need you." And, how beautiful to be needed.

—JOHN KNUTSEN
*TEN YEAR SURVIVOR*

The same day I was told I had leukemia, I found a Gideon Bible in my hospital room desk. The first verse I flipped to was, "Why do you worry, oh ye of little faith, and then He rebuked the wind and calmed the sea." Another passage read something like, "I lift up my eyes to the hills where cometh my strength."

I asked God then and there to take over my life and, if it was His will, that I be able to defeat the cancer. Even though I felt at that moment I might not have long to live, a sort of peace came over me and it has helped me through my illness.

Today I am keenly aware of what all cancer patients are going through, and here is my simple message: If you are fighting cancer at this moment, know that you are never alone. Know that I and many others are praying for you.

—JIM WEATHERS

When I was diagnosed with prostate cancer, I was discouraged because I thought of Walter Payton and his great physical prowess and wondered what chance I would have, being much older and over-weight. I began researching the various treatment options and what would be the best. It was confusing, but I decided on HDR Brachytherapy at CTCA in Tulsa.

At CTCA they taught me about the Brachytherapy so I could feel involved in my own treatment, but also stressed the nutritional and naturopathic programs that would help me. And they also talked about the importance of a strong faith in God. It was very calming and brought a great awareness to me. It is now two years since I was diagnosed and I continue to do very well. I am cancer free and a very lucky person.

—GEORGE MACIEJEWSKI

When I was diagnosed with stage IV colon cancer, I thought the worst. But I have a wonderful international family who was praying for me. One daughter-in-law is from Singapore, one from Australia and two from the United States. When I visualized their prayers circling the globe for my recovery, I felt so loved and cared for. I believe those prayers saved my life through my oncologist who was determined to keep me alive. After four years and many surgeries, treatments and procedures, I am able to do all the things I enjoy. I like to call myself the "comeback kid."

—ELLEN STEELE

Attitude is very important when fighting cancer, and so are cheerleaders. In 1991, I was diagnosed with prostate cancer. I had to drive 63 miles each way five days a week for 33 treatments. During this time I worked five hours a day and continued to bowl and dance. I was pretty tired by the end of each week, but I kept up my sense of humor as best I could. Through it all, my sister Betty cheered me on—and what a difference that makes. Two weeks ago, I had my yearly checkup and my doctor told me good-bye—I would not have to see him again. Thank you, Betty!

—PETER DANNENBERG

Family is powerful. Prayer is powerful. But when you put the two together, now that's *really* powerful. There's no question that my family and prayer got me through my bout with ovarian cancer. I praise God every day now. I look forward and never backward. Since 1990 I have volunteered 92,000 hours at Midwestern Regional Medical Center, and my advice to everyone I meet is, "Never give up hope!"

—POLLY FRIEDAY

Inspired by the unwavering faith of my family and friends, my own faith in God was restored and strengthened. Always know that He will not give you more that you can bear. Always know that He is looking out for your best interests, and no good thing will He withhold. Knowing this, what should you be doing? Take your attention off your troubles, doubts and worries. Place your entire focus and energy and God's love on the battle, and you can achieve more than you ever imagined.

—CHERYL E. BUILTEMAN

strongerthancancer

I was diagnosed with prostate cancer 13 years ago and a dear friend led me to Proverbs 4:20-23. "My son, attend to my words; incline thine ear unto my sayings. Let them not depart from your eyes; keep them in the midst of your heart. For they are life unto those that find them, and health (Medicine!) to all their flesh." God's word is strong medicine, stronger than cancer, and it's working in my life.

—ROY COOPER BEATY

When I learned I had cancer, I thought it was the end of the world, but it was merely an introduction to a whole new world. I quickly learned how much others could care, could give love, and could give of themselves. I learned that finding courage in the seemingly most difficult of times gives one dignity and character.

God gives us gifts in unusual ways. When I needed Him most, He taught me strength, love and patience—all while battling cancer. He taught me how to care, and how to value others. Be open to God's gifts in your life, too, for in the midst of your battle He is always there, always with you.

—MARTIN BERKOFSKY

Shortly after I was diagnosed with breast cancer in 1987, one of my best friends and her family went on a trip to the southwest. Throughout their trip I received postcards from every stop they made, with an encouraging line from each member of their family. It's amazing how much power, energy and good cheer can be delivered to a cancer patient on a simple 4"x6" postcard. Their thoughtfulness and encouragement was so meaningful to me at this difficult time.

—BARBARA DEANE STEIN

One weekend while I was away, a work party came and blitzed my house and garage, cleaning them top to bottom, even washing my laundry. When I was down with radiation fatigue, friends provided meals, babysat the kids, and sent all kinds of cards and flowers. I finally realized that treatment was not just about avoiding pain and making my tumor go away— it was about enjoying and savoring friends, family and LIFE!

—RAMONA P. WEAVER

strongerthancancer

If someone offers to help, take them up on it.  People
are unable to receive chemo for us, but they can
cook a meal or take us to an appointment.  These
gestures become important to both the giver and
the receiver.

—DEBBIE DUBBS

When someone asks, "Can I help?" be BOLD and
say, "Yes please!"  When our church friends asked if
they could bring us meals, I accepted.  As a family
with two teenagers, we needed our regular mealtimes
to connect during this stressful time.  We enjoy
lingering at the dinner table, sharing our thoughts and
laughing together.  Thanks to our church friends, the
question wasn't, "What should we make?"  Instead it
was, "Whose recipe are we experiencing today?"

We thought fondly of the ones who lovingly prepared
the nourishment for our bodies and souls.  We realize
we were emotionally, physically and spiritually fed by
their support.

—SARAH COOPER

You may have to fight a battle more than once to win it.

—MARGARET THATCHER

I have been diagnosed with cancer TWICE! No one should ever have cancer once, let alone twice. As I wondered how I would get through this second ordeal, my family and friends slowly formed an imaginary circle around me. They held me tight and wouldn't let anything that wasn't constructive enter this circle of life. Everyone began volunteering to help, and I am on more prayer lists than I could ever imagine. Each time I had a conversation with them, I could literally feel their strength and courage being absorbed by my body. Some days, I felt like I was draining them dry.

It is through their understanding, patience, caring and love that I am able to keep on fighting each day. My mom used to say, "God never gives you more than you can handle." It's true! Of course, I do still allow myself five minutes every day for self-pity, but God sent me so many angels on earth that I could never give up.

—ELAINE BRUCKNER

As a five-time survivor of cancer, my advice is to keep looking ahead, take one day at a time, and set short-term goals at every stage. Even the smallest goal achieved is cause for celebration, as it brings you one step closer to recovery. A piece of advice from my daughter: "The family needs to quickly move past their own feelings of discouragement and focus on making life together as comfortable and normal as possible."

—FLORRIE USATCH

I once got a card that showed a teddy bear sitting on the floor with some of its cotton hanging out. It said, "Ever feel as if you've had the stuffin' knocked out of you?" I loved that card. A recurrence of cancer feels like that. But remember, our most-loved toys were often mended more than once.

Yes, but what if the second diagnosis is worse than the first? I've had Stage One and Stage Two patients tell me that they are not so sure they could handle Stage Three or Stage Four. Trust me, if you've dealt with cancer at any stage, you have all the tools you need. You just don't know it beforehand.

—VICKIE GIRARD
*THERE'S NO PLACE LIKE HOPE*

strongerthancancer

> Birds sing after a storm; why shouldn't we?
> —Rose Fitzgerald Kennedy

Recently during the CTCA Celebrate Life event one of our administrative assistants celebrated her five year anniversary of being cancer free. We all did something special for her because this is a great accomplishment and we all saw the battle she fought and won! At the Celebrate Life event a tree is planted for each five-year survivor, and they are now on their way to planting an entire forest. Sometimes I think we focus too much on what cancer can do, and this living forest will be a visual reminder of what it cannot do!

—LINDA MORLEY

Both my mom's parents waged repeated battles with cancer. They were wonderful grandparents in every way, and their spirits still echo in my world every day. In my most quiet moments, or my moments of greatest frustration, I often hear Grandma whisper, "Believe," followed by Grandpa smiling and giving me his old familiar "thumbs up." I feel their love, courage and humor, I know they are with me, and I do "believe". . .we are stronger than cancer.

—STEPHANY WOLFF

> There will come a time when you believe everything
> is finished.  That will be the beginning.
> **—Louis L'Amour**

Always get a second opinion.  Six years after my wife died I met a new friend and decided to date again.  Shortly thereafter I was diagnosed with prostate cancer.  My doctor recommended surgery, but my friend insisted I talk to a doctor who had a new procedure.

My friend and my church prayed for me to be healed. We also believe God uses doctors to heal.  My second doctor recommended Brachytherapy and radiation.  I played golf a week after the therapy and went back to work while I was receiving radiation.  It has been about four years and I am cancer-free.  P.S. My friend is now my wife.  We were married right after my treatment.

—RICHARD BRUNSON

My sister, Beverly, was diagnosed a year ago.  After six months of treatment with her local doctor there was no progress.  She never wavered in her faith that God would heal her and came to Cancer Treatment Center of America in Tulsa for a second opinion.

strongerthancancer

Our prayers were answered on June 13, 2002 when she was told the tumor was gone. There was never a time Beverly thought she would die from this disease. Her persistent, positive attitude and faith through the eight months of treatment were so contagious, it was easy to be a family support member.

—LOREE STEFFEN

Nine years ago I was diagnosed with bladder cancer. Local doctors told me I must have my bladder removed immediately. No words can describe the despair my wife and I felt, and then a little miracle occurred.

A dear friend was taking her husband to Cancer Treatment Centers of America in Tulsa on Monday. I called CTCA and asked if they could possibly get us on the same plane—and they did! At CTCA we were treated like family. That was nine years ago and—guess what—I still have my bladder and am now cancer free!

—JOHN RENE' DIAZ

I am 71 and have two little insights for everyone. First, do not get upset if your radiologist has you back for more tests. In 1999, when I went for my mammogram, the radiologist (Dr. Kathy Wyant of McAlester, OK) called me back three times for more X rays. I was really disgusted because I thought all she was seeing was a previously diagnosed fibrocystic disease. I finally agreed to the biopsy, still thinking, "What a waste."

It turned out I had breast cancer that had already metastasized to 22 lymph nodes and was in my bone marrow. If Kathy had not been thorough, I don't know what would have happened to me.

My second piece of advice is to pull together with family and friends and fight with all you have. My family and I were devastated. Dr. Nevinny told me it was very serious, but he would treat it, and that gave us hope. Treat it he did, and my cancer has been in remission three years now. My life is back to normal, and I pray that yours will be that way too.

—BEV REDDEN

strongerthancancer

In 1995 I was diagnosed in Arizona with stage-four breast cancer. I was told that the cancer was too advanced for any treatment. They suggested I return home and call Hospice.

One month later I happened to tune in to the Trinity Broadcasting channel and heard Dr. Patrick Quillin, a noted cancer nutritionist. His lecture was simply entitled, "Beating cancer with nutrition," but what an eye-opener!

My daughter called the CTCA clinic in Tulsa and they arranged for air travel within two days. I arrived at Tulsa April 5,1995, received treatment for nine weeks and then returned every three weeks for a week of chemo until December 1995.

Proper nutrition—feeding my own immune system—remains a huge part of the treatment. I have been in remission ever since. I enjoy life every day and thank God every day for the Cancer Treatment Center of Tulsa.

—EVA JOYCE RESLEY

Because I'm a chaplain, I encourage patients to put their God between them and the cancer. I believe there are only three stages on the journey to defeating cancer: reaction, acceptance and spiritual growth. I urge all patients to move quickly to acceptance, saying, "Yes, I accept that I have cancer, but I'm going to go on living despite the cancer."
—REV. JIM FISHER

There's a lot of pressure for patients to be positive "all the time," but even people who don't have cancer aren't positive all the time. Friends and family, please remind your loved ones that it's okay to feel whatever they're feeling. Don't waste valuable energy worrying about being positive "enough." Use that energy to fight the cancer!
—ANDREA GILBERTSON

Sometimes patients have the wind taken out of their sails when they experience side effects or unexpected additions to their treatment. They interpret these events as "steps backwards," when in fact they are more like hurdles in a race. The patient and health care team merely need to jump over them. The reality is that while jumping over the hurdle, we are still moving forward…to the eventual finish line which is a cure.

—RICK JONES, RN

Wherever you go, nurses are the unsung heroes of the cancer brigade. They are the ones who provide "just what the doctor ordered," and so much more. They can fix a broken stitch, or mend a broken heart. I know, because I had a nurse mend my heart several times during Walter's illness.

From day one, Walter and I were embraced by his nursing staff. I know it had nothing to do with Walter's status as a professional athlete. Those nurses could've cared less about football—all they cared about was ensuring that Walter and I had everything we needed to remain calm, comfortable and well-informed. That was such a blessing to us because nothing is worse than not knowing "why" things are being done. Whenever Walter or I had a question, his nurses would stop right there and listen—not just with their ears, but with their hearts. Please know that I will never forget you!

—CONNIE PAYTON

My church friends had a wonderful "Tide Will Turn" party for me and everyone brought handmade signs that I still keep in my study, including: "Sure, there are ebbs and flows, but remember the tide always comes back!" And my favorite: "When you get in a tight spot and you feel that you can't go on, hold on—for that's just the place and the time that the tide will turn." The tide did turn, and I have been cancer free for two years.

—JANET CHARDIN

Our doctors don't give patients timelines, they just say they're going to do everything they can to help. God is the only one who knows our individual timelines, so no one else should be deciding yours for you. The truth is, every person is unique, so our care is uniquely structured for each person.

Family is such an important part of that care. For family and friends at home, always remember that your loved ones with cancer are still the same people they've always been. They just have a new problem, and your love will help them solve it.

—SANDY GRASSER

strongerthancancer

> The best way out is always through.
> **—Robert Frost**

Here's how I beat my Stage 3 inoperable lung cancer:

- ❖ Decided with my husband that I would beat the cancer.

- ❖ Found the best medical care I could, in a setting that made me feel valued, where they would treat me for a cure no matter what.

- ❖ Ignored unfavorable statistics.

- ❖ Got professional help and advice on all other facets— diet, psychological and spiritual issues.

- ❖ Prayed. Exercised. Drank water. Prayed again.

- ❖ Read Bernie Siegel, Vickie Girard, Greg Anderson, and Patrick Quillan.

- ❖ Joined an on-line support group. Accepted and enjoyed the love of family and friends.

- ❖ Made time to heal. Found my passion (singing and painting) and incorporated it into my daily life.

Today I'm in complete remission, living an active lifestyle that includes singing, watercolor painting, and activities in my church. I'm praying for you. You can do it!

**—KATHLEEN HOULIHAN**

# Courage comes and goes.  Hold on for the next supply.

—THOMAS MERTSON

I've been battling colon cancer since 1995. In December, 2001 my doctor in Appleton, WI, said it had spread to my liver and there wasn't anything else he could to for me. My friend Sue encouraged me. She told me not to quit. I don't know how to quit. I came to CTCA and they gave me hope.

A recent scan showed that my tumors are shrinking. I can honestly say that I came to the best place. You can live with cancer, and you can be happy if you let yourself. I want to live. This is a battle that I didn't choose, yet I'm part of the club, I'm a fighter and I make the best of it.

I've been told that I'm an inspiration. That's the good that comes from the cancer. I try to enjoy my life. You can't think about cancer 24 hours per day. You rely on your family and friends, and they help you through it. You don't know what you have inside until you're tested. Sometimes the weakest person can be the strongest.

—LINDA FAIRCHILD

> Take good care of yourself, just as you have taken such good care of others.
> —**Dan Zadra**

It's always amazing to watch adult children (some with gray hair themselves) come to the treatment center and try to "parent" their own parents. "Did you eat your vegetables today, Mom?" someone will scold. They so want to care for their parents, just as their parents cared for them all these years. Before long, however, the children usually relax. They begin to realize that, yes, nutrition is extremely important, but most patients do their best in that department and would much rather fill their visits with smiles, and the sharing of wonderful parent/child memories, and loving emotions.

—SUSAN PEREZ

I'm a nurse. Both my parents eventually died of cancer, but we learned many things together along the way. I realized early on that it was difficult for us to talk about cancer, surgery, chemo and everything that goes along with it, so we created our own "vocabulary."

My parents loved to travel and had taken some wonderful trips together, so Mom and I decided to use travel as our new metaphor. We envisioned Mom in an antique car (Dad had several), traveling down a dusty

strongerthancancer

country road toward a distant destination. The car
was moving slowly and as it traveled along it became
harder and harder to see the point of departure. Mom
saw a bright sunny road ahead and would describe
Dad waiting with a big picnic lunch.

Using this image, Mom and I could finally talk in short-
hand about where she was in the process. I would ask
her where her Model T was each day, and she would
answer, "stopping for gas" (meaning she needed a
bite to eat), or "cranking it up" (meaning she needed
to change position).

We had decided on a code, and I knew that when she
said "rounding the bend" she would mean it was time.

On a Sunday afternoon with the entire family together,
she smiled and said softly, "I'm rounding the bend."
She died later that evening, but she died on her terms.
I learned many things from my mother. In our last days
together, I learned to speak a new language with great
clarity. It's a language that cancer doesn't understand,
and can't comprehend—a language of love, hope, faith,
dignity and courage. I am so thankful.

—MARCIA PETERSON

> Count each day a separate life.
> —Seneca

My father was a patient at MRMC for the past three years with advanced colon cancer. The Oncology staff at MRMC were honest about his disease, and yet gave him ALL the possible treatment options available. Even when his disease was not responding to treatment, they never gave up and offered him the choice to decide what the next step would be. This approach gave my father and our family hope and strength to fight his disease.

A lot of life can be packed into three years. Dad was a craftsman who built cedar strip canoes. After his diagnosis he was able to finish one canoe, build another and build one kayak. He died on June 11, 2002, but his ability to continue what he loved, and the time our family was able to spend with him was a priceless gift.

—CAROL LEPPER

While fighting ovarian cancer, I shared this with my support group sisters to put those night fears to rest: "Grasp today with all your might, it's the tomorrow you feared yesterday."

—LINDA SMITH

strongerthancancer

About two years after my father was diagnosed with colon cancer, I was devastated to learn that my husband wanted a divorce. My son and I immediately went crying to my parents. Despite his own burdens, my father held out his arms to us and said, "I'm here, I will always be here for you." I remember thinking, "Oh Daddy, if only that were true."

Now that my father has passed away, I think back and realize it really was true. Dad is still here for me, and will always be here for me. He taught me so much about life. Many times I stop to think what Dad would say and do in certain situations—and I immediately feel his presence, strength and advice. My husband and I did not divorce, after all, and we are happier now. My father left such an impression on us, including our deep conviction that nothing is stronger or more important than family.

My father chose treatment at a remarkable clinic in Zion, IL and I know it gave us more quality time together. Today I am a Colon Cancer Alliance volunteer in his memory.

—NATALIE PORTER

Deep down,
you know things will
probably come out
all right, but sometimes
it takes strong nerves
to watch and wait.

—HEDLEY DONOVAN

> The best thing about the future is
> that it comes only one day at a time.
> **—Abraham Lincoln**

Believe in your heart that cancer is not a death sentence, but a life experience that you will one day look back on and actually treasure in certain ways. The suspense is difficult, I know, but have faith that everything will work out for you, and it usually does.

—PAM M.,
*6-YEAR OVARIAN CANCER SURVIVOR*

When our daughter, Jenny, was diagnosed at the age of 20, we were overcome with emotion. On the day Jenny had surgery, a nurse handed us a note with the words, "One day at a time" written on it. Just five little words, but they have been the most helpful to our family.

—JANE SUHR

This passage by Elizabeth Janet Gray was passed on to me and has been a wonderful reminder: "Sorrow cannot be fought and overcome; it must be lived with. Somehow we must learn not only to meet it with courage, which is comparatively easy, but also with serenity, which is more difficult, being not a single act but a way of living."

—ROBERT J. BERAN

107

I need to take an emotional breath, step back,
and remind myself who's actually in charge of my life.
**—Judith Knowlton**

Don't rush into surgery or other treatments. Take the time to get a second opinion, even if you have to pay for it out of pocket. Cancer is a baffling, multi-dimensional, irrational and non-linear disease. There's no one sure-fire cure or way to fight it.

Take some time for you and your family to get centered and find out your options before you commit to one path. It feels terrifying and overwhelming at first, but eventually you will know what you want to do.

Then plunge into your treatment with all your heart and soul.

—STACEY DENNICK

I was diagnosed in April, 1999. For two days I was worried I wouldn't have time to prepare for my death. Then I took a deep breath and asked God to give me more time for my husband and family and friends who needed me. From then on I had no fear, and I felt a sure faith that I would be cured. I am 74, and this I know with all my heart: With God, prayer, positive

strongerthancancer

We all live in suspense from day-to-day; in other
words, we are the hero of our own story.
—**Mary McCarthy**

thinking, loving friends and family, and good doctors,
we really are stronger than cancer.

—JERALDINE M. WARE

Two days after my prostate cancer consultation with
my doctor, I decided to view cancer as an opportunity instead of a problem, and I have been blessed
every step of the way.  Here are the changes:

- ❖ Decided to lay my burden at the foot of the cross.

- ❖ Let God be my strength in fighting cancer and found
  happiness in watching Him do it.

- ❖ Tried new foods.  Told my wife that she had been right
  all along about green vegetables.

- ❖ Learned the facts about nutrition and supplements in
  strengthening my immune system.

- ❖ Freely gave and received encouragement.  Shared my
  faith with others.

So far, at least, every problem really has shown itself
to be an opportunity to improve my life and health.

—RON MARTIN

> May your burdens be lighter and
> your star shine even brighter.
> —**Earl Graves**

Here is my simple formula for keeping a
positive attitude:

- Relax
- Let Go
- Let God do His job

—CARIN HANSEN

Keep hope alive at all times, believe in a positive
outcome, lean on your family and friends, and take
God with you on the journey. As Bob Moawad says,
"Never put a period where God has put a comma."

—DONA DAVIS

These words from the Sanskrit had special meaning
for me during chemotherapy, and I hope other cancer
fighters might enjoy the spirit: "May the long time sun
shine upon you, its healing warmth surround you, and
the light from within guide you on your way."

—DONNA RUFENACHT

strongerthancancer

**H**ave faith!  A good friend sent this piece of prose to me.  I do not know the author, but it's been such a help over the last five years: "Faith is the bird that feels the light, and sings while the dawn is still dark."
—VIRGINIA STARKSBERRY

**T**his little prayer was said often during treatment and is still a daily comfort: "Lord, remind me that nothing is going to happen to me today that You and I together can't handle.  Amen!"
—CORRINE DESHAIS

**T**hink of the cancer cells as intruders and visualize yourself kicking their butts.  Then pray.  Don't be afraid to ask for help from friends or family.  Pray some more.
—CONNIE RACHAR

**M**y favorite little poem for you and yours: "Sad soul, take comfort, nor forget, the sunrise never failed us yet."
—GEOFF WEINRICH

As soon as healing takes place, go out and heal somebody else.

—MAYA ANGELOU

I'll be honest with you, I am a very private person, but when I finally walked out of that hospital, cancer-free, I couldn't wait to tell the whole world that it can be done!

—JOHN OLIVERA

Celebrate your conquests, both large and small. Within one cancer battle there are many individual success stories—first steps taken, fears faced and conquered, tears shed and dried. Starting today, celebrate them all! Success stories are food for our hearts and souls. Success stories should be shouted from the highest rooftops: "I beat it! I beat it! I beat it!"

By sharing success stories, you help destroy the monster, slay the dragon, and send the bully called cancer running for all of us. It is not enough just to defeat cancer. No, we must tell others and share our victories so that others in turn will not be so afraid to fight. Success stories save lives.

—VICKIE GIRARD
*THERE'S NO PLACE LIKE HOPE*

> We can only be happy now, and there will never be
> a time when it is not now.
> —**Gerald Jampolsky**

When I was going through treatment, my friends and family started bringing angels. They brought angel cards, Teddy bear angels, and other angels. These angels made me feel good. Receiving them from friends and family brought me closer to God and I wasn't afraid. I had a feeling that these angels were keeping an eye on me.

Then one day I got this idea. What if each us just did something small to help in the fight against cancer? It would all add up. I'm good with ceramics, so I turned to my husband and told him that I was going to make ceramic angels for children with cancer. I made 30 and took them to the hospital the next week, and gave them out to the kids.

It broke my heart to see these children so ill. They had the sheets pulled up over their noses and when I pulled an angel out of the box, the sheet dropped down and their little eyes got real big. They smiled, and every one of them said thank you. This made my day. I knew right then and there that I had to keep making these angels for them. So far I have given out more than 200 angels and the kids call me the Angel Lady.

—LORI STUMPF
*COURTESY AMERICAN CANCER SOCIETY*

strongerthancancer

Faith and family have gotten me through my bout
with cancer. It's difficult, but you just have to have
hope, and take one day at a time. If you think about
it, that's what we're supposed to do anyway, whether
we have cancer or not!
—BARBARA HIPPLEHEUSER

Having cancer did indeed bring my family closer.
My sister was right there through every procedure
and always giving encouragement. My husband
called me almost every evening that I was away and
was right here to help and support me when I came
home. My daughters called and kept in touch to
make sure I was okay, always checking on me and
bringing things to cheer me up or just making a meal
so I didn't have to cook. They also kept an eye on
my husband while I was gone just to be a support.

One more thing I might add is that when my church
family began to pray, they simply did not let up. I
cannot tell you how much it has meant to me and my
family just to know of all the prayers and the support
from our church. God love you all!
—BEV REDDEN

> Believe there's light at the end of the tunnel.
> Believe you might be that light for someone else.
>
> **—Kobi Yamada**

In 1998 I had breast cancer surgery and reconstruction at Johns Hopkins. My prayers were answered and the results have been excellent! I have since made multiple trips to Europe with my husband and am doing wonderfully!

I am a quilter and I wanted to give something back. And so, along with other volunteers, we quilted the Hopkins Quilt of Encouragement. With all 63 squares filled with breast cancer survivors' signatures, the quilt hangs in the Hopkins Breast Center to send a bright colorful message to all new patients and their families: Yes, together we are winning, we are stronger than cancer.

—MARIE JOHNSON

While receiving chemotherapy I read the following advice from a compassionate physician, and I now share it with all newly-diagnosed breast cancer patients who call the Helpline at Living Beyond Breast Cancer:

"I have come to realize that my patients can live with the word 'incurable,' but they cannot live without the

strongerthancancer

> In the deserts of the heart,
> let the Healing Fountain start.
> —**W. H. Auden**

word, HOPE! What every patient needs from friends, family and physicians is a ringing endorsement of HOPE—and the constant reminder of the truth. The truth is, no matter what the odds may say about a particular type of cancer, those odds are being beaten all the time."

—RENEE BERNETT

Cancer is a disease that affects the whole family, so it just makes good sense for the whole family to come together and fight back. I was diagnosed five years ago at the age of 39. My diagnosis became a "family diagnosis" immediately. I was lucky enough to have a wonderful, supportive husband, and my parents also put their lives on hold and helped me get through the rough spots. I understand, now, when people say there are blessings in cancer. We were a close family before the diagnosis but our relationships and our love were made even stronger by this disease. I thank God daily for my family and their love.

—UNSIGNED

Here is the test to determine whether your mission on earth is finished: If you're alive, it isn't.

—RICHARD BACH

During my treatment, I realized that I couldn't
completely count on fixing myself. I had to let go of
my fear and let God and family do their part, too. I
figured, "I'm still here, so my work on earth must not
be over." It's when we think that we might be at the
end of our abilities that God's possibilities are just
beginning.

—VIOLET JONES

My favorite thought during treatment came from a
close friend who had gone through a bone marrow
transplant: "I know things happen for a reason. I
know this is probably just a bump in the road, not
the end of the road. And I know God is probably
just teaching me a life lesson, but couldn't He have
taught me the same lesson with a flat tire on I-96?"

—MARY ELLEN SMITH

Everyone knows what the pink ribbon represents.
I wear mine proudly and thank God daily. Be
determined to stand with us, the living testimonials
of this once-feared disease!

—DAISY LAY

Keep a daily win book.
If your life is worth living, it is worth recording.
—**Marilyn Grey**

Keep a daily journal. Participate in support groups and, above all, keep looking ahead and planning future events.

—SHARON SAVAGE, 10-YEAR SURVIVOR

Becoming a cancer patient can be a crash course in learning how to ask for what you want. People care and WANT to help us win, but they don't know how, and many of us don't know how to ask!

Keep a journal—I call it a "treasure map." Each morning write down what you want from this day. Then give yourself permission to aim for it, and if you need help, ask for it! Cancer centers offer all kinds of support that you might not be aware of, including therapists for you or your family to connect with, and even rides to your doctor appointments. Don't wait until you and your family are worn out; find out early what your resources for support are, and then learn to ask!

—JUNE GREEN

strongerthancancer

**K**eep a journal. If you go through a period where there seems to be no progress, look back to where you were a month ago, or six months ago. I could always find a change. Sometimes there had been much more progress than I realized.

—CAROL MAATA

**Y**ou are the first and most important partner in your healing. Self love, journaling, positive self-talk, imagery and affirmations are all ways to bathe yourself in love. Blend together with the love and support of family and friends, and you are definitely stronger than cancer.

—LINDA SCOTT

**M**y advice to every family is to keep a journal. I lost my dad to pancreatic cancer when I was only 16. Through a brutal one-year battle he never gave up, never complained (at least to me) and always found joy in the simple things in life, and in our time together as a family. I kept a journal through that entire year and it gave me comfort then and wonderful memories now.

—KIM SWIERENGA

Suppose your friend or loved one is going for an extended hospital stay. What kind of a gift could possibly bring them joy and inspiration every single day?

When I was about to start my second bone marrow transplant—twenty-one days in the hospital—I received a big basket. It was from my beloved nurse and friend, Mara. Inside the basket were 21 gift-wrapped packages of all shapes and sizes. She had sent instructions to open one each day in the sequence in which they were numbered. She said they were "nothing special"—just some treats to brighten my day—but, oh, how important those gifts became to me and my family!

Each day would bring the question, "Have you opened your present yet?" It became a production, something to look forward to. Regardless of what else the day held in store for me, my basket from Mara held the promise of a pleasant surprise, a gift of love meant just for me. It mattered not whether it was a crossword puzzle, hand lotion, a book of

If you had five minutes to live,
who would you call and why are you waiting?
**—Michael Nolan**

inspiration or something as simple as flavored lip gloss. Each and every one touched my heart and made me smile.

As the basket neared empty, and the pile of gifts dwindled, my days in the hospital, too, were drawing to a close. Finally the last day came. As I sat in my room, waiting for my "get out of jail" papers to arrive, I picked up the very last gift. What could it be? I excitedly tore off the ribbons. How absolutely perfect: a box of sparklers to celebrate my "day of independence from cancer treatment!" Believe me, no big-city Fourth of July fireworks finale could have ever made my heart soar more than the sight of those little golden sparklers. Thank you, Mara, for loving me and caring about me.

And to you, Dear Reader: If Mara, and I, and Connie Payton, and all the people at CTCA could bring just one gift to everyone reading this book, it would be these golden words: "Have faith. Be not afraid. Be hopeful. Together, we really are stronger than cancer."

—VICKIE GIRARD

Dear Connie Payton,

I know you lost Walter, and how much it must hurt.

I am only 12, and I lost my grandmother in April.
I called her Grandma Lela. People say I was her
favorite, but I knew it wasn't true. There's three of
us grandchildren—me, age 12, Brandon, age 9, and
Bradley, age 6. We all love her, but I was her only girl,
her only granddaughter.

Connie, I miss her so much and still cry, but I've
gotten through it. The night she died I was on my
way home from Alabama, and it's like she waited until
I was home to pass. My friend, Angela Perridotto's,
father passed away the night before, and Angela
and I support each other. I'm a cheerleader, a
softball player, and a band member. This stuff helps
me get through it too! I hope you and your children
are being strong.

Bye Connie. I think your husband was a really
nice man.

**—BRITTANY SEXTON**

Walter's illness helped our entire family realize how
we take so many things for granted.  Once he knew
his time was short, he wanted to do everything as
a family.  We played together, and prayed together.
Walter and I found ways to get away and be alone.
Taking long rides in the car with me driving—now that
was really something—because, if you knew Walter,
you knew that he was quite certain that no other
person in the world could drive as well as he could.

Walter and I were blessed with some truly great
friends.  (You know who you are!)  Hearing your
voice on the telephone or having you around to
lend a helping hand, to laugh with or to cry on your
shoulder, meant everything to us.  Walter had friends
who would come to the house and get him right out
of bed to go play a practical joke on another friend.
Cancer or not, you knew that Walter was still Walter
and, no matter what, friends are still friends, and you
never let him forget it.  From the bottom of my heart,
thank you, each and every one.

—CONNIE PAYTON

AMERICAN CANCER SOCIETY
A nationwide, community-based not-for-profit organization dedicated to providing the public with cancer information and resources. ACS has listings of events and programs both nationally and locally:
800-ACS-2345
www.cancer.org

CANCER RESOURCES
An on-line guide about specific types of cancer, treatments, and cancer-related information, services and organizations:
Cancer Resources
457 West 22nd Street, Suite B,
New York, NY 10011
Phone: 1-800-401-2233
Fax: 212-243-1063
info@cancerresources.com
www.cancerresources.com

CANCER SOURCE
An interactive site devoted to providing complete and current information on all types of cancer for patients and loved ones and medical professionals. Also offers information about special programs and coping with cancer:
www.cancersource.com
info@cancersource.com

CANCER TREATMENT CENTERS OF AMERICA
With hospitals in Tulsa, OK., and Zion, IL, and clinics throughout the country, CTCA offers compassionate, world-class care for cancer patients and their families. By involving patients and their

families in every aspect of the treatment process, CTCA seeks to empower patients and utilize commonly overlooked complements to traditional treatment, such as nutrition, spirituality and psychoneuroimmunology:
www.cancercenter.com
1-800-234-0509

CANCER TREATMENT CENTERS OF AMERICA at Midwestern Regional Medical Center:
1-800-615-2955
1-800-577-1255

CANCER RESOURCE CENTER
Gurnee, IL,
800-940-2822

CANCER FIGHTER HOTLINE
1-800-765-9920

CANCER TREATMENT CENTERS OF AMERICA at Southwestern Regional Medical Center:
1-800-788-8485
1-800-773-0273

CANCER TREATMENT RESEARCH FOUNDATION:
By sponsoring the world's most innovative and promising clinical scientific research, CTRF gives cancer patients and their families hope for a cure. Ninety-nine percent of every dollar donated goes directly to cancer research:
www.ctrf.org
847-342-7450
1-888-221-CTRF (2873)

CENTER FOR MIND-BODY MEDICINE
A not-for-profit organization dedicated to combining modern medicine and ancient healing traditions. Directed by Dr. Jim Gordon, a leader in the field of mind-body medicine, the center addresses the mental, social, emotional, physical and spiritual aspects of health and illness:
Center for Mind-Body Medicine, 5225 Connecticut Avenue, NW, Suite 414, Washington, DC 20015
Telephone (202) 966-7338
Fax (202) 966-2589
www.cmbmorgcenter@cmbm.org
www.cmbm.org

CHILDREN'S CANCER WEB:
A national not-for-profit organization that provides a directory of information about types of childhood cancer and resources for children living with cancer:
www.cancerindex.org

OFFICE OF CANCER COMPLEMENTARY AND ALTERNATIVE MEDICINE
A division of the National Cancer Institute, OCCAM coordinates the research of and provides information about complementary and alternative medical practices such as acupressure, acupuncture and nutrition:
OCCAM,
National Cancer Institute, NIH
Executive Plaza North, Suite 102
Bethesda, Maryland 20892
888-NIH-NCAM (644-6226)
www3.cancer.gov/occam

WALTER PAYTON CANCER FUND
Connie Payton and her family established this fund in June 2000 to give cancer patients and their families hope for a cure. Ninety-nine cents of every dollar donated goes directly to cancer research:
www.payton34.org
888-221-CTRF (2873)

RECOMMENDED BOOKS

BEATING CANCER WITH NUTRITION
By Patrick Quillin, Ph.D., R.D., C.N.S.
www.4nutrition.com
800-247-6533

CHALLENGE CANCER AND WIN!
By Kim Dalzell
www.challengecancer.com

HOW TO PREVENT AND TREAT CANCER WITH NATURAL MEDICINE
By Dr. Michael Murray, Dr. Tim Birdsall, Dr. Joseph E. Pizzorno, Dr. Paul Reilly

THERE'S NO PLACE LIKE HOPE
By Vickie Girard
www.compendiuminc.com
800-914-3327

# IN WALTER'S MEMORY

❖

From my family to yours, I hope you find a special place
in your home for this book. Take it with you on your
journey and always remember that knowledge is power.
The more we learn about cancer, and the more we share
our personal stories with each other, the faster we will
make the future safe for our children.

To that end, my children and I established the Walter
Payton Cancer Fund in June of 2000. WPCF is committed
to clinical research that delivers immediate treatment
options and genuine hope for a cure. This is part of
Walter's living legacy, and I know he would be proud of it.

True, Walter lost his battle, but no one ever really loses
to cancer. Let his legacy and this book remind us that,
"Cancer's shadow can never extinguish our love. It cannot
suppress our faith. It cannot restrain our hopes. It cannot
destroy our compassion. It cannot end our friendship.
It cannot tarnish our memories. It cannot silence our
courage. It cannot conquer our soul. And it cannot
vanquish our spirit."

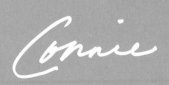